FROM F*CK NO TO F*CK YES SEX!

ANGELA SKURTU, M.ED.,
LMFT-S, ACST-S

A Special Thank You

There are many to thank for the creation of this book. Anya Overmann helped me to clarify my thoughts and ideas. Whitney Stubblefield illustrated the picture in chapter 1. Addie Sanders helped me create the picture on the back of the book. The following beta readers read through my book and offered edits and various ways to shape the content--- Julie Noyes, Greyson Smith, and several unnamed beta readers who are rock stars and my cheerleaders. My husband listened to me talk for *countless* hours about my ideas. Finally, my daughter inspires me every day to write this information. She's 10 this year and learning about her own body. Every day, the lessons I teach her are lessons adults need to learn to improve their mind/body connection. Finally, for countless other people who shared ideas, business strategies, and pushed me to publish, thank you. Thank you all for being my supporters, family, and friends.

Table of Contents

Introduction 1

CHAPTER 1:
Demolish Your Sh*tty Mental Real Estate 7

CHAPTER 2:
Upgrade Your Mental Real Estate, Elevate Your Sexy Life........... 28

Endnotes 47

About the Illustrator 53

About the Author... 54

About the "Open Bedroom Doors" Book Series 56

Introduction

"I give you hand jobs in the shower!" Shannon, a 65-year-old woman screamed at her husband.

"Yes, but you're too rough with it! You need to be gentle! Tickle the balls a little," Greg, her 70-year-old husband pleaded.

"Hand jobs" was the topic in my office for about an hour on a cold, gray Tuesday morning. They had been married for 40+ years. Shannon was tired of having sex and hoping that this part of her life would be over by now. Greg was not dead yet! He had hoped at this time- retired with adult kids out of the house- they could rekindle their old flame. This was proving a difficult task. Like many other couples I help, they had dwindled into a sex-starved marriage. When they did have sex, it was lackluster at best.

I'm Angela Skurtu and it's my job to professionally turn people on so they *want* to F*ck each other. I'm a Sex Therapist. I help couples who are best friends who have *friend zoned* each other take their relationships from F*ck No to F*ck Yes Sex by teaching creative sexuality and normalizing conversations about sex. I wrote this book series because sex for too many people has become a problem. Every day, I find myself having similar conversations with different people. Many of the skills I teach are repeated again and again. By reading this book and the books to come in my *Open Bedroom Doors* book series, you will learn how to get the passionate sex you desire.

You Deserve Great Sex!

Sex and desire are not magical experiences only few lucky people get to enjoy. They are the result of behaviors- skills that over time can be trained, learned and embraced. They are the result of comfort in one's body and skin, comfort with a partner, and comfort to experiment in a safe environment. I'm a Certified Sex Therapist and Supervisor (AASECT), Licensed Marriage Therapist and Supervisor (AAMFT), keynote speaker and author of two books, "Helping Couples Overcome Infidelity: A Therapist's Manual," and "Pre-Marital Counseling: A Guide for Clinicians." I've been teaching couples since 2008 to have better sex, rekindle their romance, learn to orgasm, find their passions, and have fun in the bedroom. By the end of this book series, you will know how to do this too!

There's a reason you aren't getting the sex you crave. Maybe you had zero sex education growing up. Maybe you learned about sex from friends, from porn, or through trial by fire. If either case is true, you have likely had the same type of sex repeatedly across many years. Add to that, people rarely talk about their sex lives. So, you don't know how they are keeping their sex lives strong. What are the steps? What kind of communication needs to happen? The pages of this book are a window into the world of good sex. Specifically, this book is going to change the way you think about sex.

In the media, we see various displays of sex. In a typical

situation, a man grabs a woman and flings her across the bed, kissing her body quickly as he rips her clothes off. She is equally involved in ripping off his clothing and kissing passionately. Their bodies both deeply breathing and heaving as they thrust into the throes of romance. Both of their faces looking upwards as they orgasm gracefully and forcefully together. But what if what you see on TV is not what you're getting at home? What if you don't want to rip your partner's clothes off and you aren't getting those magical orgasms? You might feel like something is wrong with you.

You do not need to turn into some prototype of desire seen on TV, found in movies, books, or any other form of media. Quite the contrary, I want to give you permission to become your unashamed, authentic sexual self-whatever that means to you. You will find yourself going from F*ck No to F*ck Yes Sex.

Who is this book for? I work with couples who are best friends. You are good to each other. You enjoy spending time together and you are partners in life. You are great at talking through many of life's issues, but one issue continues to cause problems—Sex. You do everything else right! For some reason, you have *friend zoned* each other. It started out sexy. You remember being romantic at some point. What changed?

With this book, I help best friends who have *friend zoned* each other transform your sex life from F*ck No to F*ck Yes Sex by changing the way you think about sex. We all have some weird stories about how we learned about sex. Some of you had families that avoided sex like the plague. Other parents may have given you a book to read by yourself, but you weren't allowed to ask questions. Or if you're like me, you were raised in purity culture and taught pretty shameful messages about sex. Regardless of your sexual origin story, you likely have developed negative messaging around sex that limits your ability to enjoy sex with your partner.

With this book "From F*ck No to F*ck Yes Sex," and with

my *Open Bedroom Doors* book series I will transform your sex life by teaching you creative sexuality and normalizing conversations about sex. As you walk through this journey with me, you will change the way you *think* about sex and so you can *enjoy* better sex.

How can you most effectively use this book? It is loaded with information, tools and ideas for changing the way you think about sex so you can start having quality sex. You can read the book solo or with a partner. Included in this book series, you will find references to my YouTube channel and my podcast where I offer free skills and strategies about sex.

A few years ago, I was sitting in a conference room at a networking luncheon. The teacher asked us to come up with one line describing what we do. The people around me brainstormed and chatted. I sat there nervously. *How do I describe to people what I do? It's a business setting! Can I even say sex in here?* I nervously fidgeted in my seat.

"What do you all think about 'I open bedroom doors?'" I cautiously asked. I had already introduced myself earlier to the table as a couples and sex therapist.

"I like it," a woman next to me replied. "Why don't you test it with the bigger group?"

The speaker asked for participants to share their taglines. I boldly raised my hand. *I hope I don't get kicked out of here! If I'm going to go down, I might as well go down in glory!* He called on me.

"I open bedroom doors!" I called out to a group of over 500 people.

"You've got my attention," the speaker replied. "And what do you do?"

"I'm a Sex Therapist!" I replied. The audience roared with laughter and a camera person randomly clicked my picture. From then on, the tagline stuck. That is what I do every day. I open the bedroom doors of couples around the world who want to have passionate sex again. I believe we need to talk about sex and treat it like a casual conversation. Sex shouldn't be locked up in a room like this shameful, dirty thing. It's a natural, healthy part of your life.

This is the first book in the *Open Bedroom Doors* book series. The book series will tackle a variety of sexual challenges that couples and individuals face. It's not sex that's complicated. It's your *relationship* with sex that is complicated. With this book series, I'll help you develop a healthier relationship with sex so that you can enjoy the great sex you deserve.

I also have included information from many of the sex therapists before me who have written amazing work and informed my writing. Without their knowledge, I would not be where I am today. Sex therapists Esther Perel, Paul Joannides, Laurie Mintz, Emily Nagoski, Wendy Maltz, Kathy Labriola, Ian Kerner, Michael Metz, Barry McCarthy, David Ley and many others have all inspired me. I humbly and gratefully appreciate their work in the field of sexuality and all its done to inform the ideas in this book.

The stories in this book are true. I have altered the names, information, and any identifying features of the people to protect their confidentiality. However, I have tried to keep their words and conversations as close to their original meaning as possible.

Why so many "f*cks," Ange? When you see the word "f*ck" in this book, it has multiple meanings. I refer to love making and to hard-core F*cking. I use F*ck as my term playfully, respectfully, assertively and hopefully. Because when it comes down to it, you are likely reading this book because you want to learn to f*ck and to enjoy f*cking. "F*ck" is our plain language. It is one word that has multiple meanings. A common way I sign books is, "A good F*ck goes a long way." Because it does. No other experience like a good F*ck is so memorable and so valuable. I hope in this book, you will enjoy a good f*ck and learn to have many more good f*cks on your journey!

Join my email list at **Openbedroomdoors.com**

CHAPTER 1:

Demolish Your Sh*tty Mental Real Estate

Sex starts in the mind. Sex begins with your thoughts and how you think about sex. To have good sex, you need a healthy mental outlook on sex. I had a client couple, Greg and Melissa, who were having the same sex every week. I call this type of sex an "arrangement." Once weekly, at the same time, in the same place, they would have the same sex. It would start Sunday morning. They woke up in bed, warm in the covers, eyes still sleepy. He would lean over to her and start kissing the back of her ear. Melissa thought to herself, "Here we go again." She would feel that familiar pressing of his erect penis in her crack. Then as he rubbed her breasts and kissed the back of her neck more, he would slip inside her and they would have penetrative sex. Melissa was getting bored with this routine. They did it because it was familiar sex, and they knew it worked. However, it was getting dull. Melissa would dissociate through much of it.

I asked Melissa about her thought "Here we go again."

"At that point, I stop paying attention and just let him do his thing," Melissa replied.

"You go to Neverland?" I asked. She looked at me, puzzled with a smirk. "Have you ever tried something different?"

She eyed me curiously, "What do you mean?"

"You know you have a choice, right? You can continue to do what he typically likes. Or, you can take action and do something you like. Did you know you could take the reins?" I asked.

She stared at me bewildered. "I guess I assumed I had to do what he wants to do."

"If you were to take the reins, what options could you take in that moment? Give me three things you could do as soon as you think 'Here we go again.'" I asked her. An eerie silence filled the room as she contemplated. I refused to give her these answers!

"I guess I never thought I could take control. I could . . . grab his hand and put it somewhere else?" I think to myself, *she's not sure of herself yet, but she's getting there.*

"Absolutely! That's a great answer. Tell me another one!" I replied.

"I could turn around and start kissing him or I could tell him to do something different," she replied, seeming more confident.

"Exactly! There's no right answer here. You could do any number of things. But the one thing you have to do is stop being passive. Don't simply let him do what he wants without having a say for yourself. That's the death of your desire for sex," I added.

This book will help you change your thoughts about sex so you can have great sex. As a Sex and Marriage Therapist for nearly 20 years, I have dug into the minds of hundreds of individuals and couples around the topic of sex. The way you think about sex truly impacts the way you enjoy sex. If you think sex will be good, you are more likely to be fully engaged in the sex, ask for what you want, and communicate with your partner about your needs, wants and desires. If you think sex is bad or negative, you are more likely to shut down or even dissociate during sex. Your thoughts about sex impact your relationship with sex. Sex is not a dirty word. It's a natural part of a healthy relationship. This book will teach you how to change your thoughts so you can have good sex.

Brain Real Estate

Think of your brain as real estate. Your brain has a limited amount of real estate that can be occupied by thoughts. People, things, and ideas compete for your attention. For example, when you are on Facebook, every time you get an ad telling you to buy products, that company is competing for your attention. In fact, marketing companies spend a great deal of money hoping to take up as much of your brain real estate as possible. It happens every day with TV, radio, social media, and video games. To dig in and explore your sexuality, you need a safe space in your brain to do so — you need to free up mental real estate so there's space for fun.

Some people's brains have become unsafe for healthy sexuality. That lack of safety can result from trauma, body or sexual shame, severe anxiety, being raised by abusive people, or any number of other reasons. If every time you think about sex, your mind goes to a dark place, then currently your brain is not a safe place for enjoying sex. Basically, for you to be sexual or comfortable in your sexuality, you need to feel safety in your mind, body, and context.[1] This first book will teach you to create safety in your mind.

Imagine a beach resort. You are walking through the resort, and it is meant to be relaxing, calming and soothing. However, as you walk, you notice there is construction going on. Suddenly, instead of the ocean waves, you hear loud, aggressive noises. You think you can get past this and still enjoy yourself, but then you notice someone left tools, broken glass, and even some sheet rock on the path to the beach. You must walk very far around it to even get there. Again, you try to move past it, but the more time you spend at this shitty resort, the harder it seems to enjoy the beach and *actually* relax.

For many of you reading this book, your brain feels a lot like this sh*tty resort when it comes to sex. You want to relax and enjoy sexual encounters, but there are a lot of obstacles in your way. For example, when you get naked, imagine body image issues as the construction noise. You are trying to relax, but your mind keeps saying, "I'm fat! My stomach looks funny. Don't let him see my stomach." You try to distract yourself from these thoughts, but then other thoughts pop in like, "Did I do the laundry? Did we turn off the kitchen lights? Is the garage door closed?" We could consider these thoughts as the broken glass on the path at the resort. The more these thoughts compete for your attention, the harder it is to really enjoy the sexual experience.

It all boils down to negative messaging that takes up too much mental real estate in your brain. To enjoy sex, you need to take charge of your brain real estate and free up space for safety. Some readers won't have a safe space when they start this book, and if you're one of those readers, that's OK. This strategy of freeing up mental real estate creates not only a safe space in your mind but also a *fun* space.

How Thoughts Can Impact Your Relationship with Sex

"My vagina is icky. I hate my smell. It's disgusting."

"I'm not good looking enough for sex."

"I've past my prime. I'm too old!"

"I'm not a sexual person."

The previous statements are examples of sexual criticisms[2] or negative sexual thoughts — based on ideas and preconceived notions for what sex "should" mean. If you don't measure up to your own idea of what sex "should" mean, it will shut down your sexuality. Basically, if thoughts like these take up your brain real estate, your brain is not a safe place to be sexual. Without safety, there is no space for fun or creativity.

In <u>Come As You Are: The Surprising Science that Will Transform Your Sex Life,</u> Emily Nagoski talks about desire as a form of curiosity[3]. When you criticize yourself, you shut down the process of curiosity. Nagoski uses the phrase "don't yuck my yum." This means don't put down people's desires or sexual interests. I want to shift this phrase to "Don't yuck your *potential* yum," or "Stay Curious." There may be pleasure in sex you haven't discovered yet. An example of "yucking your potential yum" in action is when you're watching a show. A sex scene comes on, and your first reaction is, "I would never do that!" or "That's gross!" This is "yucking your potential yum." If you've never tried the thing you saw on TV, you honestly don't know what the experience would be like. You may feel scared to try it, but criticizing the scene gets you no closer to finding out if it would be fun. I invite you to *stay curious* when you learn about different sexual options. *Stay curious* doesn't mean you have to try everything you learn about. It means you ask questions. You keep an open mind.

If you see a couple spanking each other on a show, stay curious and ask yourself:

"What does this couple get out of this experience?"

"What can I shift about this to make it fun for me?"

"Would I spank my partner or would my partner spank me?"

"What intensity would make spankings fun? Harder, softer, more playful?"

"Are there other body parts you can spank, or does it have to stay on the butt?"

When you ask questions and stay curious, you learn ways you could explore your relationship with sex to make it more fun. If you're watching this show with your partner, try stopping the show and asking each other questions like these. Stay curious and have a conversation. This is how you avoid "yucking your potential yum." Consider different acts and get comfortable with a variety of ideas. Talk directly, openly and casually about these ideas with your partner.

Desire is Not a Switch. It's a Thermometer.

Many of you have been taught to think about desire as a light switch that is either on or off.[4] *What turns you on? Find his turn ons and turn offs.* This is not how desire works. A better way to think about desire is in terms of a thermometer. Essentially, when more negative thoughts take up real estate than positive thoughts it keeps you at the colder end of the thermometer. Initially, you can work towards having more neutral thoughts about sex. Then, you can work on creating more warm or hot thoughts (that is, if you want to).

F*ck Yes — F*ck No!

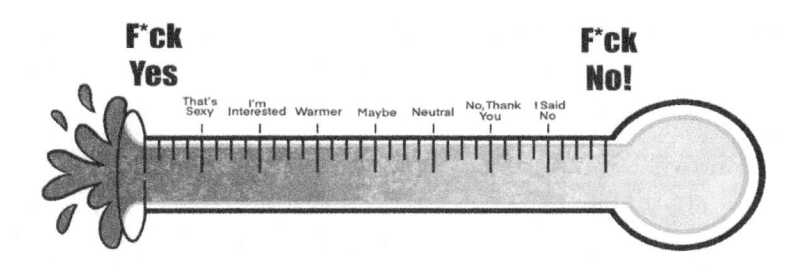

That's Sexy | I'm Interested | Warmer | Maybe | Neutral | No, Thank You | I Said No

As you can see from the diagram, the Desire Thermometer goes from "F*ck No" to "F*ck Yes." There is a spectrum of "no" spaces, a spectrum of "maybe" spaces and a spectrum of "yes" spaces on the thermometer. When our brains are filled with negative thoughts around sex, you'll notice you stay cold towards sex or certain aspects of sex. It becomes harder to move into a yes space around sex if most of your mental real estate is filled with shame, guilt, trauma, hurt, anger, or any other negative thoughts around sex. There are many spaces between F*ck No and F*ck Yes. You may find it's much easier to move towards the "Maybe" spaces first.

The middle spaces or the "Maybe" spaces are spaces of sex neutrality[5]. If you think of curiosity as the "Maybe" space, your goal can be to move towards the middle---to remain very neutral and non-judgmental towards sex. In fact, you or your partner may actually exist in a position of neutrality around sex. You don't think positive or negative thoughts around sex. You simply see sex as a thing people do. That's still a step in the direction towards "F*ck Yes." It is easier to go from sex being neutral to positive than it is to go from sex being very negative to very positive.

On the upper end of the thermometer are the spectrums of yes. Even looking at the higher end, not everyone thinking about sex is at a "F*ck Yes." Sometimes people are at a place of sure or why not? Some people will start a sexual experience when they are in a "Maybe" space and grow into more of a yes or more of a no.

There is a spectrum to experiences that are yes, maybe and no---and when you learn to move through them, it creates freedom and the ability to enjoy sex.

"But what about people who really seem to turn their desire on like a light switch?" Many of my clients have argued with me. "I can literally walk by naked, and he'll be hot and ready to go!" I would argue this partner is already riding high on the Desire Thermometer for any number of reasons. If your brain real estate is filled with positive sexual experiences, you are already resting higher on the thermometer. Perhaps you stay in the "Maybe" space all the time. I truly believe when clients stay in neutral to positive zones around sex, then it becomes easier to go from neutral or warm to hot. You have a shorter distance to go to hot if you stay warm all the time. However, if in your brain, sex stays in a very cold space on the thermometer, you have further to travel to get to "turned on."

When you realize there is a spectrum of ways to think about and experience sex, it becomes easier to try new things and learn how to enjoy different sexual acts. You also learn that desire is not about turning each other on or off. You learn to turn "up" the heat and keep it warm daily in your brain and possibly in your relationship. You may have never tried anal sex before---giving or receiving. If you never have had an experience with it, you may have uncertainty, but until you have actually tried it, you don't know if it is a good experience or not. If you approach it thinking it will be bad, you will likely have a bad experience because you won't learn enough about the experience to make it enjoyable.

If you approach sexual acts with curiosity or neutrality, you may take time to learn about doing anal sex properly. You will learn that lube helps it feel better and that if you warm up the rest of your body first, then the experience will be nicer. You will likely ask questions about what positions make it fun and safer. You will feel more open to learning to relax your sphincter muscles. You may start with a finger to get used to the sensation of something penetrating your anus before using something bigger like a penis or dildo. Even with all that knowledge, you will need practice and experience before it will feel good. You will likely make mistakes as you learn to enjoy anal sex, but that's part of the journey.

In many books, videos and articles, experts encourage positive thinking.[6] I regularly see that it's difficult for most of my clients to move from negative to positive thinking. They simply don't believe the positives. One time, I suggested my client, Janna, go home, stand in front of a mirror and start saying positive things about herself every day over the next week. We're sitting across from each other in my office.

"What happened when you tried looking at yourself in the mirror?" I asked Janna. She avoids eye contact and adjusts in her seat.

"I just kept seeing all the things I hated. I tried saying that I was beautiful like you said, but I didn't believe it. All I could see were my flaws and I ended up having a fight with myself and quitting a few days later," she replied. I think to myself, *What is wrong with Janna? Why can't she just be nice to herself? Am I doing something wrong?*

With my mind sufficiently blown, I realized that going from negative to positive is impossible for some people. They need a middle ground. As the Desire Thermometer shows above, there are middle spaces or "Maybe" spaces that are neutral. People don't easily make huge leaps from one type of thinking to another. They need steps! Once you realize there are smaller steps in between, you can learn to move one or two steps forward.

"So, you feel like you're gaslighting yourself? I never thought about it like that before!" I replied to her. "How about you work on staying neutral with your intervention? Instead of saying positive things about your body, let's say very factual things about your body. Here are some examples. It has curves. It is colored pink in some areas and peach in others. It has a top, bottom, and middle. Can you practice looking at your body in the mirror every day and saying neutral things about yourself and see what happens?"

Wouldn't you know it, the next week she came in with "some" success. To be fair, we had to work on neutral thinking over the course of several months. Changing negative thought patterns doesn't happen overnight. The first week, she came back and explained she could do neutral thinking for a minute or two, but she would still go back to the negative. I encouraged her efforts and made sure she gave herself credit for these small, valuable steps. Janna was never neutral about her body so the fact that she even did it for a short time was a huge accomplishment. Over months of practice, she was able to maintain neutral thinking for longer and longer periods of time.

Back to the Desire Thermometer. Then you are thinking about sex or body image in a more positive way, stay realistic about what you can do. If you look at the thermometer like a train station, there are many stops along the way from "F*ck No" to "F*ck Yes." Humans are a lot like trains at the zoo. We are slow moving. This isn't like the subway train where you zip from one area of the city to the next in a matter of minutes. Human behavior change takes time. You are more likely to move from "F*ck no" to "no, thank you" then you are to move from "F*ck No" to "F*ck Yes." Please be kind and patient with yourself as you are learning this new way of thinking. The long-term goal is to create a daily space of neutrality around all sexual acts. That type of thinking takes time and patience.

To put this in perspective, let's consider how you think about oral sex. What's your inner monologue about oral sex? Do you say,

"I don't like oral sex, it's not for me?" Stay curious with yourself. Where does this message come from? Did you have a bad oral sex experience in your past? Have you seen oral sex depicted in a positive way that might inspire giving or receiving?

Some of you have seen oral sex depicted in a grotesque way through porn. Picture the typical image of a woman going down on a guy and gagging. Was the woman's face clearly not enjoying the sexual experience? And if that image of oral sex was all there was, I could understand why it would be a "F*ck No!" on your Desire Thermometer. Who would want to gag or have their head shoved into a penis like that? If you own a penis, who would want to make their partner gag or feel discomfort like that? You want your partner to enjoy giving you oral sex-not suffer through it.

People who enjoy giving blow jobs don't do it that way. They may make out with the penis like they are kissing any other part of the body. They may use their hand cupped around the penis with their mouth to make the experience feel better for themselves and their partner. They show love to the penis with their mouth. If they do enjoy the practice of deep throating, they have practiced with a partner who was respectful and gave them opportunities to explore it in their own way without any pressure. If you see oral sex can look more positive as I have described, you may shift how they think about giving or receiving a blow job. You can check out my video **"How I Wish People Talked about Oral Sex,"** on my YouTube channel for further instruction here **YouTube.com/@AngelaSkurtu**.[7]

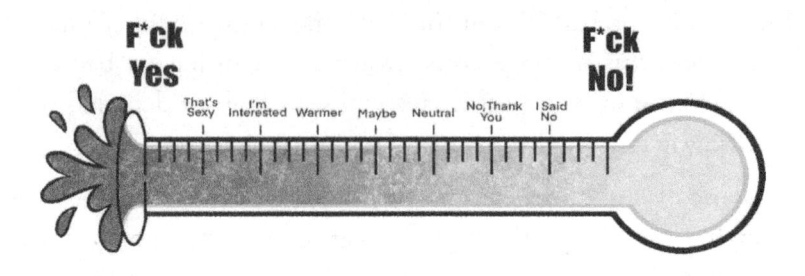

Look at the Desire Thermometer again. You can't immediately move from "F*ck No" to "F*ck Yes." There are stops along the way and humans move as slow as molasses. If you to change your view of oral sex, you could start by thinking about it neutrally, then move to a "Maybe" spaces, and then move to a "yes" space. You might imagine your mouth and head close to a penis until you regularly thought about a penis neutrally. Once you have more neutral thinking about the penis, you may practice laying your head next to your partner's penis on a regular basis. You would need to ask your partner to be a willing participant and let you control the situation. Maybe you would do this while you watch TV. In your head, you would practice neutral thinking such as, "This is my partner's penis. It is round. It is next to my head." I know it doesn't sound sexy, but we aren't aiming for sexy first. We're creating neutrality and comfort. In your brain, you need to feel safe before you can feel sexy. This process is actually called exposure therapy.[8]

Over time, you might practice putting your partner's penis near your mouth or in your mouth but in slow ways that feel neutral--- a peck here, a kiss there, light strokes with your tongue. Stay neutral in your mind. You may think to yourself, "It's my lips on skin. It's my tongue. I choose how to use it." Practice staying open-minded and curious. The longer you do this, the more neutral the action will become. Once a sex act becomes neutral, you can begin thinking about oral sex in more fun, enjoyable ways.

Remember brain real estate? Every time you neutralize a different sex act or sexual thought, you remove sh*tty homes or resorts in your neighborhood. You can't simply go from a broken-down neighborhood to a lovely, renewed neighborhood. You have to intentionally tear down the homes and real estate that is taking up space. You may need to spend some time reworking the soil and the grounds. You have to rebuild some foundations.

What Impacts Where You Land on the Desire Thermometer?

It's not sex that's complicated, it's your relationship with sex that is complicated. One basic thing that impacts your interest and desire for sex is safety in your mind, body, and relationship context. If you have a lot of negative sexual thoughts, you will likely land closer to the "F*ck No" space on many sexual acts such as oral sex, penetrative sex, finger sex, sensual massage, etc. Negative sexual thoughts can include perfectionism, binary thinking, sexual criticisms, comparison thoughts, emotionally self-abusive language, trauma, shame, and negative body image. Contrarily, positive thoughts such as self-compassion, cheerleading thoughts, encouragement, appreciation, gratitude, love, and healthy body image will likely put you on the "F*ck Yes" side of the thermometer or at the very least, the "Maybe" space.

While we aren't focusing as much on the body and your relationship in this book these two also do shape how we feel about and desire sex. If in your body you feel relaxed and comfortable around sex, then it is easier to stay more open to and interested in sex. If in your body, sex feels painful or uncomfortable, it will be harder to desire sex. Also, if you are in a relationship that is caring, loving and supportive, it is easier to desire and want sex. However, if you are in a relationship that is unhealthy or abusive, over time you will desire sex less. I will discuss the body and the relationship context in future books, but for now, let's stay focused on the mind.

If your goal is to shift from "F*ck No" to "Maybe" or from "Maybe" to "Why not?" then you need to analyze which of these thoughts are taking up mental real estate in your brain and then make a conscious decision to shift this thinking. In the following sections, I will describe the negative thought processes getting in the way of your sexual desire.

1. Perfectionism or "Be Your Best!"

Perfectionism[9] is commonly known in the sex therapy world as the death knell of a good sex life. It is thinking that in order to have sex, everything needs to be perfect. You need to shower because you can't have any smell at all! Also, you need to shave and you can't have a single hair on your body. Wait, you also have to brush your teeth, floss, mouth wash, and then maybe you can get naked in front of each other. But wait! There's more! You have to have a great date night where nothing goes wrong! You have to get dressed up, look your best, smell your best, act your best and feel so incredibly romantic that you swoop each other up in your arms and make magical love! Oh yeah, don't forget the magical sex part. The sex has to follow a perfect formula. You build hot energy. You fall into bed without hurting each other and you both are completely turned on and ready to F*ck each other's brains out. Sounds reasonable right? Wrong!

The problem with perfectionism sex is it's not real life. Let's paint a picture of what sex actually looks like! You wanted to go on a date, but it's Friday night at the end of a *very* long week. Both of your brains are fried from working long hours. Then you get home and your kids miss you and want your attention. You cancel the babysitter because neither of you is really feels up for getting dressed again. Instead, you watch a movie with your kids. It's Friday, so they ask if they can stay up late and--- because you both miss them--- you cave. You finally put your kids to bed at 10:30pm. Now you have "us" time but you're both tired. You decide to cuddle and make a plan to get sexy time with each other in the morning. The next morning you wake up, avoid any kissing because you have NOT brushed your teeth. You smash into each other's genitals, somewhat asleep and somewhat awake. It feels pretty good. One of you orgasms first then gets out the Hitachi vibrator to give the other one an orgasm. Then you start the next day with your kiddos. And that's only if you're good at following through with your sexual goals!

If you want to have good sex, you do have to let go of the idea that sex needs to be perfect, because it's not perfect. It's messy. It's silly. It's weird. It can feel good. It can feel good enough. It can even feel "meh." People who keep their sexual expectations too high will end up being constantly disappointed with their sex lives. Or, they will avoid sex altogether because it is never good enough to follow through.

Sarah and Jason were struggling with sexual perfectionism when we worked together in sex therapy. Sarah had previous partners who were a little more skilled lovers but they were terrible people. She had finally found in Jason an awesome partner. They were best friends and shared everything together. However, Jason was a little sexually shy and not as skilled as her previous partners. Sarah genuinely loved when guys would take charge and show confidence in the bedroom. Whenever Jason showed even the slightest bit of hesitation, Sarah would get angry with him. This exacerbated his problem. He got into sexual perfectionism by avoiding initiating sex with her unless he knew he was doing it exactly right. But it was never perfect. He could never show the right enthusiasm or have the right timing because again, her need for it to be perfect made it more likely for him to make mistakes.

To be fair, Jason and Sarah had to work on a lot of things to get better with each other in the bedroom. But to specifically work on perfectionism, they needed to learn how to embrace chaos and make mistakes more fun. Put simply, they had to create a safe environment to fail. In fact, one of the ways they learned to do this was by intentionally having shitty sex and learning to enjoy it. If you struggle with perfectionism, you are going to have to make some conscious choices about how to enjoy a variety of sexual experiences whether they are perfect or not.

2. Binary Thinking

Binary thinking[10] is when you make decisions that are black and white. There is only all good or all bad. You can either be left or you can be right. There is no room in between. Desire is not a switch. You are not "on" or "off." Desire is a spectrum. There is a spectrum of "yes," a spectrum of "maybe" and a spectrum of "no." If you only think about sex in the form of "I'm turned on" or "I'm turned off," you miss a lot of wiggle room in middle.

This binary thinking is not solely focused on desire. There's a lot of binary thinking people engage in. Another type of binary thinking is body dysmorphia[11]. You are either beautiful or ugly. Fat or thin. Mr. America or Sasquatch. There can only be one body type that is the right one and if you do not possess it, you are wrong. Again, this binary thinking causes extraordinary harm. Think about it. If everyone is supposed to look one way, then virtually none of us should be sexual and we all should hide in a shed to protect the children from our hideous selves. It's not a fair way to think about yourself, is it? And yet, we do it every day!

Another binary is spontaneous sex versus responsive sex. In her book, Nagoski discussed these in the following way[12]. There's spontaneous sex in which the interest in sex just hits you. Boom! You are ready to have sex and you are interested. That is spontaneous sex. Then, there is another type of desire which is responsive desire. When you are responsive, you experience desire in response to cues. You have brakes that shut down your sexual interest and you have go pedals that rev your engine. Even this idea is too binary. You are either responsive or spontaneous.

When I talk to my clients about these two desire types, they often challenge me. For example, Terrence and James were in session and I discussed the two desire types. "You see, if you are responsive, you experience desire in response to cues. But you also have brakes that can shut down your sexual desire. So you are working on reducing your brakes and maximizing your go pedals," I said explaining the different desire types.

"Can you be both?" Terrence asked.

"What do you mean?" I asked.

"Well, I feel like at times I can feel spontaneous where it just happens and at other times, I can have brakes. I don't feel like I fit into one desire type," Terrence replied.

"I also think I can do both. I was more spontaneous in the beginning of the relationship and now that we've been together for a while, I am more responsive. Can you change over time?" James asked.

"I don't know. I guess you can," I replied.

"You know, come to think of it, I have been different types at different times in my life, too," Terrence chimed in. I have had this conversation many times with multiple couples. I have learned that even the two desire types are too binary. Desire is more nuanced than that. Desire is a type of spectrum. Your tendency to be more spontaneous can shift with new relationship energy[13] versus long term attachment. It can shift with your hormonal cycle. Some women will say they feel more spontaneous during ovulation and more responsive at other points in their cycle. It can even shift

23

with age. Some male clients have said they were spontaneous in their younger years, but now at 60+ they find themselves more responsive and needing a deeper connection.

Another sexual binary is penetrative sex versus foreplay. Foreplay might be considered every sexual thing you do other than penetration. But what if you want to have oral as your main entree? What if fingering is the fun sex act? What if making out is the fun part of sex for you? What if your favorite type of sexual act is spending long hours storying a wild sexual fantasy and it doesn't even include touch?

When people use binary thinking to describe sex, they severely limit themselves. In general, when you use binary thinking in most aspects of your life, you severely limit yourself. It is either black or white, left or right, all good or all bad. This type of thinking is a cognitive distortion,[14] and it essentially ruins your life. The world is way more complex! We need variety and spectrums. In order to do well in this world, you have to embrace the gray zones. There are choices and outcomes. There is a spectrum of outcomes, but ultimately you have to keep moving forward and learn from the choices you make. To live in this world successfully requires you to embrace complexity. To truly enjoy sex requires you to see beyond penetration and embrace creative sexual expression.

3. Sexual Criticism

"I'm just not a sexual person. I'm not pretty enough. I'm too old."

Brene' Brown calls this voice the "inner critic[15]" and I like to call it "the judge." You can also call it "the narcissist" or "monster." Sexual criticisms are mean language you use to describe yourself, your body, your sexual identity or your sexual feelings. They can include absolute language, "You always say no to sex!" or "You never enjoy sex." They can include character assassinations.

"You're not a sexual person!" or "You are frigid." Another version of a character assassination, "I'm the problem. It's all my fault. If I wanted to have sex, we wouldn't be in this mess." These sexual criticisms put the blame solely on yourself and block your ability to move forward or change your behavior. To be fair, we might call these various versions of self-abuse.

One unique thing to pay attention to in yourself is to listen if you use "You" language or "I" language in your inner monologue. "You" language can sound like blame and can be a sign you have taken someone else's criticism and internalized that monologue within yourself. If a partner blames you for the relationship's sexual problems or if a parent said accusatory things to you growing up about sex, your inner critic may use "you" language. If you use "I" language such as "I'm just not wired like that," or "I'm not a sexual person," you may be engaged in fixed mindset[16] talk which is a type of mental block that holds you back from growing. If you notice any of this sexual criticism in your inner monologue, start by curiously noticing when and how this language shows up.

4. Comparison Thoughts

"Why am I not like this person? Why am I not this way when my friend is this way?"

"I'm not as pretty as her."

"I'm not as sexual as my friends."

"I wish I were like you. I wish I could just want sex."

Comparison thoughts[17] are when you compare yourself to others in a way that puts you personally down. Recently, I had a colleague who was doing a speech on sexual health. If I am in a good mindset, then I will say to myself, "I am so proud of his accomplishment. It is amazing he is getting to speak about a topic he loves!" My inner monologue is one of gratitude for the other person and genuine pride for him. If I am in comparison thoughts, I might think something like, "Why does he get all the good speaking engagements? I try and I try but I never get to his level. What am I doing wrong?" This type of comparison mindset is the start to shame spirals for me personally. There are similar sexual shame spirals that my clients experience as a result of comparison thinking.

Comparison thinking commonly shows up when you look at social media. Rarely do people post a picture of themselves falling in mud unexpectedly. They post a cute birthday picture here and a sweet vacation picture there. When you mindlessly scroll, your mind starts to subconsciously believe that this is what people look like and their lives must be magical. Then, over time, there can be ways you look at yourself and say, "Why don't I look that pretty?" This comparison mindset is just another way we put ourselves down internally and ultimately reduce our connection to reality.

5. Emotionally Self-Abusive Language

"Really? You are leaving the house looking like that? You are so ugly and disgusting. You don't deserve to go out in public looking like that."

"Sex is gross."

"What's wrong with you? You can't do anything right!"

"You are such a whore! (insert explicit self-rebuke)"

"You're worthless!"

Emotional self-abuse is the kind of emotional abuse[18] that you may have learned by someone else doing it to you, then you started doing it to yourself. Essentially, when you grow up in an emotionally abusive household, you learn to internalize that emotionally abusive language and use it on yourself. If your inner critic is shaming, blaming, criticizing, guilting, humiliating, ridiculing, dismissing, accusing, neglecting, or verbally berating you, you are emotionally abusing yourself. Emotional abuse takes up a *lot* of brain real estate. And when your brain is full of all that shit, there's little room for fun, sexy stuff!

When you are sexually abused, these triggers will feel like a whole-body experience. A trigger[19] is a stimulus that can cause old memories and/or a physical reaction to occur. An example of a trigger could be a certain smell or song that was present during an abusive episode. In the present, when you hear that song or notice that same smell, your whole body reacts in fight/flight/freeze/fawn as though you are going through that trauma again in the present. Even though you may simply be driving your car to work or doing laundry.

While we will talk more in depth about trauma triggers in the chapter on emotions, any negative or abusive self-talk you have internalized as a result of sexual abuse, physical abuse or emotional abuse in your past can impact your ability to stay present for your sexual experiences. Sexual abuse essentially creates a minefield of triggers in current sexual relationships. For more information visit my YouTube channel and watch the video, "How the Body Protects Itself from You," at YouTube.com/@AngelaSkurtu.[20]

CHAPTER 2:

Upgrade Your Mental Real Estate, Elevate Your Sexy Life

In the previous chapter, we discussed various types of negative thinking that get in the way of an enjoyable sex life. In this section, you will understand to change this for yourself. Essentially, you need to root out the old sh*tty homes and resorts of negative thinking and make room for newer homes and resorts that are *way less* judgmental and have better construction. In this section, we will cover cognitive change mechanisms to root out unnecessary negative self-talk. Keep in mind that these negative messages have been living in your brain for a very long time. The skills I describe in this section are meant to become "a practice," not a onetime skill. Internalized negative messages have likely lived in your mind for a long time. It takes diligent practice and repeating the skills over time to truly shift your mind's real estate.

Someone else cannot drag you out of the "No Space" or turn you on. You can make choices to improve your own mental real estate, but your partner cannot magically bypass your negative messages. Desire is not a switch. It's a thermometer. You must first turn up the heat in yourself before you can work with a partner to amplify sexual energy. If you personally don't move from "F*ck No" to "Maybe," and then potentially to "F*ck Yes," there is nothing a partner can do that will make it happen for you. If anything, their constant trying when you are in the "no space" will push you further into your "F*ck No" space. You must bring your own sexual energy to the table. Then, as a team, you can amplify sexual energy. No partner can drag sexual energy or passion out of you.

In this section, we will cover two skill types to impact your negative thinking about sex. The first group of skills focuses solely on going from negative thought patterns to more neutral ways of thinking. These skills include learning how to manage your trauma triggers, mindfulness, and neutral thought mechanisms. Another way of thinking about these skills are strategies to take you from "F*ck No" to the "Maybe" space. The second group of skills helps you go from neutral to positive or "Maybe" to the spectrum of "Yes" and *hopefully* "F*ck Yes" someday. These skills include self-compassion, cheerleading statements, sexual mind games and creating a safe learning environment.

1. Managing Trauma Triggers

When we become triggered, it becomes impossible to move out of "F*ck No" in that moment. It is protective. Your brain and body automatically flip into your sympathetic nervous system[21] to protect you from danger. As we discussed earlier in this chapter, when you have a certain stimulus occur like a smell or sound that reminds you of the past trauma, your whole body automatically flips into its fight/flight/freeze/fawn response and chooses how to protect you. All humans need this system to survive, and it has been instrumental in keeping you alive up until this point.

However, when you have lived through chronic trauma, your body can get more sensitive to smaller triggers when you are no longer in the traumatic environment. As a result, you may be minding your business at work and suddenly find yourself panting, tight in your shoulders, and hot in the face for what appears to be no reason. What happened? A stimulus that reminded you of that past trauma whipped your body into its sympathetic nervous system. In sex, this may happen more frequently as there are many opportunities for triggers to pop up. Perhaps there is a certain touch or sexual act that reminds you of a past trigger.

This trigger management skill is meant to help you notice a trigger happening in the moment and make a conscious decision about how to manage the trigger. Keep in mind that this is only one trauma skill. Some of you reading this may need to investigate therapy or other trauma books that bring more depth to this topic. If that's the case for you, check out "The Sexual Healing Journey," by Wendy Maltz[22] "Healing Sex," by Staci Haines,[23] or the "Healing Sexual Trauma Workbook," by Erica Shershun.[24] You can also visit Youtube.com/@AngelaSkurtu and look up "Trigger Response Cycle."[25]

Trigger Management Skill

1. **Observe** – *Consciously notice you are having a trigger*. What sensations are present in your body? Try to describe them to yourself neutrally. Heat in face. Panting breaths. Tense shoulders. Ask yourself "what" questions to become more aware of where you are in the present. "What's actually happening in this moment?"
2. **Physically Deescalate** – *Take physical actions to slow down your body's nervous system.* You can count down 5-4-3-2-1 and make sensory observations (I hear, I see,

I smell, I feel). You can take deep breaths while very slowly walking. Noticing each step you take. You can also use box breathing,[26] which is where you breathe in for 4-four counts, hold your breath for 4-four seconds, breathe out for 4-four seconds and then hold for another 4-four seconds. Imagine drawing a line with each step into a box. You can even change your location. The objective of physical de-escalation is to convince your body that it is safe again. You can take any physical action that basically slows your body down and reminds you that you are not in danger.

3. **Emotionally Deescalate** – *Internally talk to yourself in a way that soothes your system.* Talk to yourself with neutral talk or self-compassion[27] (It's okay to mess up, because you're doing the best you can. It sucks now, but maybe it will get better. I am here because I want to be here, not because I *must* be here. It's okay to not be okay. We all struggle. It's okay to fail. It's okay to make a mess, just clean it up when you're ready. It's okay to leave this mess). You will have to tweak this part of the skill to find out what works for you. What is soothing for one person might feel very damaging to another person. Think about using neutral language or the language you would use to speak to a friend in a time of need. For ideas, you can visit Youtube.com/@AngelaSkurtu and look up "How to Practice Self-Compassion," or "What is Sexual Self-Compassion."

4. **Repeat** – Repeat Actions 1-3 until if you rated your stress on a scale of 1-10, you land on 3 or below. (Special note: If your baseline of stress is a 5 on most days, then repeat until you move to your baseline of 5 out 10 on the stress scale).

5. **Return to the original activity or do something different.** *Make an intentional decision about what action*

to take next. Some triggers are easier to move through than others. If you were working and you feel like you can go back to work, then do so consciously. However, if you still feel raw after the trigger occurred, choose to do something different until you feel better again.

How to Address Triggers Over Time

Those old sh*tty homes are going to be *trouble* on their way out of the neighborhood. Most of us have had trauma for many years. As we all know, old habits die hard. As you get better at managing triggers in the moment, the next step is to work on minimizing the impact of these triggers over time. Start keeping a small log of the types of things you are triggered by. Is it a certain touch from your lover? Is it certain words or phrases? Smells? Sounds? When you are not triggered, begin to observe patterns about yourself and your triggers. When do they show up? Is it during certain sexual acts? When flirting? Do certain compliments trigger you? Stay curious and non-judgmental towards yourself.

I had one client, Amanda, who was triggered by compliments. Anytime her partner Brad would say she was beautiful, she would start a war with herself in her head. She would internally say things like, "No, you're not. You're so fat and ugly. He is just saying that to be nice." Outwardly, she would react with tension. She wouldn't say anything to her partner, but he could tell that physiologically, her body changed and closed. Over time, he stopped complimenting her because he didn't want to make her feel that way.

I discussed this reaction with her. Amanda stated she wanted to get better at receiving compliments, but she could not control the physiological response her body naturally had when she heard compliments. She worked on using the trigger management system

I described above. She asked her partner to start complimenting her more. I explained to him that Amanda would still have her current reactions, but she would be working internally on shifting the way she received those compliments with her partner. Brad was reluctant at first because he never wanted to hurt Amanda. Amanda reassured him she would be internally working through those triggers in a more conscious way.

Amanda consistently worked on shifting that internal triggering when she heard compliments from Brad. Sometimes she would ask him to offer compliments and sometimes he would do it on his own without her prior knowledge. It was important to practice moving through the triggers in multiple settings to lower the intensity of the trigger. Amanda found that she was better able to move through triggers when she was prepared at first. The longer they did the skill, the less she found herself reacting to the compliments even when she received them randomly. Over time, she stopped experiencing triggers associated with compliments at all.

What people typically do in response to anxiety is avoid the situation altogether or over control it. To manage triggers, you must gently expose yourself to the triggers in safe environment and make a conscious decision to respond consciously to the triggers over time. This is exposure therapy, and it is effective when done gently and consistently. Again, none of my skills are magic cure-alls. They take time and diligence. When you master them, you will feel as though you have mastered life in some cool way! Technically, you have.

2. Neutral Cognitive Change Mechanisms

Shame holds us back, and it's hard to shift from negative to positive. But there's an entire spectrum between negative and positive — between "F*ck No" and "F*ck Yes" — that you can work within. I call it the "maybe space," but really it is neutral, curious, and non-judgmental. In the famous words of Yoda, "Do or do not. There is no try."[28]

In sex and body image, neutrality sounds like this.

"Those are breasts."

"This is sex."

"Some people have sex."

"Sex is part of life."

"Middle parts" from the children's book, <u>Sex is a Funny Word: A Book About Bodies, Feelings, and YOU</u>[29] (This is an alternative to using the term "private parts" which implicitly sends the message that penises or vulvas are private, dirty and possibly shameful).

I'll never forget the movie scene from Mean Girls.[30] The girls are standing in front of a mirror together taking turns criticizing a body part they hate about themselves. "God, my hips are huge!" "Oh please, I hate my calves." Lindsay Lohan, the main character of the film, had never engaged in this type of self-loathing. She stared at the girls bewildered. Body image is an all-too-common issue that many people face. Alongside sex, we receive messaging around which bodies are "sexy," and which aren't. As a result, a lot of us feel terrible about our bodies.

Neutral thinking is one way to shift how we feel about our bodies and sex. Instead of thinking about sex as bad or gross or sinful, you work on seeing sex as natural or neutral. *Sex is a part of life. Sex is a thing people do. Sex is a thing I do, sometimes. My body has shapes, colors and textures.* If you listen to the language, it is neutral and does not judge anything one way or another. It simply states facts. If you have a negative inner monologue about sex, your body, or intimacy, it is virtually impossible to shift from negative or the "F*ck No" space to a positive or "F*ck Yes" space. Neutral thinking is the step in between.[31]

I once had a client, Rhianna, who hated her mommy belly so much that she could not look at it and could barely touch it. Her belly was a shameful space. She wouldn't dare wear a bikini! If her partner touched it (even accidentally during sex), she would recoil and could no longer enjoy the rest of the sexual act. That's how powerful her shame was. It stopped sex completely in its tracks. It would have been impossible for her to go from "I hate my belly," to "I love my belly." She had to work on body neutrality first. I asked this client to use neutral words like "texture," "lines," "curvy," "soft," "shape," and "peach color," to describe her belly. We practiced having her use neutral language while looking at her belly, touching her belly, having her partner touch her belly, and having her stand naked in front of a mirror looking then not looking. To be clear, it took her an entire year of practicing this body neutrality[32] before it had an impact on her ability to touch her belly or receive touch. However, the constant practice helped her to have sex again without fear or shame around her belly stopping the experience.

Some people will live the rest of their lives in shame. Some people will make it to body neutrality and that's as far as they can go. The journey is a challenging one for any person who has internalized self-criticism and self-abuse. People who chronically feel a lack of safety due to trauma can struggle to reach neutrality. This is why some people find themselves in marriages or relationships where sex is consistently not there— moving to neutral is a huge deal. If you have made it to this point or if you ever get to it after years of shame and negativity, please give yourself a win (which can include a high five or a gold star sticker). It's a huge feat to get from "F*ck No" to the "Maybe" space. I'm proud of you. If you're not there yet, I am still proud of you for starting this journey. It's hard to face these demons and yet, here you are! Amazing.

3. Mindfulness

Mindfulness[33] is the practice of being fully present at this moment--staying curious and non-judgmental. We as humans are naturally wired to judge our environment. The practice of neutrally observing things is one way to consciously challenge yourself into thinking about your body, sex acts, and intimacy in a more neutral way. Mindfulness is NOT clearing your thoughts! It is instead redirecting your brain towards neutrally observing sensations in your body, mind, or environment. In this book, we will focus on mindfulness of thoughts, but in future books we will cover mindfulness in other ways related to emotions and behaviors.

Spectrum thinking is a type of mindfulness. *I practice* every day to manage my own negative body image thoughts. Yes, you guessed it. I struggle with body image, too. Spectrum thinking is one way of challenging my own personal judgments on bodies. It all started one day when I was watching a performance with my kiddo up on stage. There were 40 little girls dancing. Some were tall, some were short, some were wider, some were littler in the middle. Each girl's skin tone was a little different. Each girl's smile looked a little different. Every girl represented body variety. Suddenly, it hit me. We're supposed to look different! Variety is the norm! Variety is beautiful, magical, special. I cried watching the girls dance and realizing the importance of recognizing this variety and cherishing it.

Spectrum thinking is the act of consciously noticing and seeing the world around you as full of variety. There are no two bodies exactly alike just like there are no two trees exactly alike. When I noticed the impact of forcing myself to not only see but embrace the spectrum in the show, I realized I needed to do that every day to remember to love myself and my own body variety.

Spectrum thinking is a version of mindfulness in which you consciously notice and appreciate the variety of life in all its splendor. You can do it by looking at trees, plants, animals, people, fruits, etc. Yes, you can look at a peach and notice it has similar traits to other peaches. Spectrum thinking is the practice of looking at a pile of peaches with mindful curiosity to notice and appreciate how each peach is varied and different as well as similar. It is the practice of truly convincing yourself that variety is the most natural part of life. It is normal and healthy. We need variety to survive in this world. Anytime I find myself comparing myself negatively to a peer, I challenge myself back into the "Maybe" space with spectrum thinking.

You may struggle with spectrum thinking at first. For example, if you own a vulva and have a negative image of your vulva, you can look up the Great Wall of Vulvas.[34] This website shows a wall of vulvas that have various shapes, sizes and looks. Spectrum thinking involves recognizing there are a world of vulvas, and that variety is the norm. Variety is beautiful. We don't need to contort and reshape our bodies and minds to look exactly like the people we see in the movies. We need to embrace our natural variety.

Another example of mindfulness is something I like to call *mental yoga*. It is the practice of noticing your sensations (inside your body or in your environment) for one minute. Sensations can include sight, smell, taste, touch, sound, balance, energy in the room, weather patterns, lighting, water, etc. You are going along in your day, and you make a conscious decision to notice one of the senses curiously and non-judgmentally. You are not clearing your mind, because that is next to impossible. You are instead redirecting your attention for a short period of time to a sensation either inside your body or inside the environment you are occupying. For examples, you can go to Youtube.com/@AngelaSkurtu and look up "Minute Mindfulness"[35] or "What is Mental Yoga and Why Should I practice it?"[36] If were working on your computer, you could stop to take one minute to redirect your attention to a sensation. As I was working on this book, I picked sound. I was sitting in my outdoor room. I directed my brain towards sound sensations. I heard my neighbor beating his outside throw pillows-*pounding, thumps*. I heard the sounds of cicadas. It sounded like *swallowed buzzing*. There was a rhythm to it almost like lifting and lowering. Birds were chirping. A *high-pitched chirp*, a *lower chirping* sound closer, a *rumbled humming*.

Notice my words. I describe the sounds, but I am not adding judgment. If I were judging I might say, "Those damn birds won't shut up!" "Those cicadas are screaming so loud!" I don't say this. I simply sit and presently pay attention to the sounds. That is an example of mental yoga. Doing this type of exercise for little minutes here and there daily will help you practice curious, non-judgmental thinking. For those who struggle with the idea of meditation, it's an easier alternative.

If you use your environment or something outside your body, you may notice energy in the room. Imagine you are in a coffee shop. For those of you who are empaths, you may walk into a coffee shop and instantly pick up on the two people who are in a fight to your left and the annoyed coffee shop owner behind the counter. You see their facial expressions and your body senses their energy. If you are using mental yoga to play with your environment, you can practice noticing these energies in the room non-judgmentally. If I am being judgmental, I might say to myself, "They are pissed at each other!" If I'm judging the shop owner, I might become people pleasing to accommodate his agitation and say, "I'm so sorry you're going through this."

Mental yoga involves noticing these energy levels without taking on the energy of the room. For a minute, you can scan the room and stay curious and non-judgmental. When you see the couple to your left, neutral engagement sounds like the following in your head: *Rising energy; Physical bodies moving; Arms animated; Faces tight.* If you notice the language, it is a challenge to stay neutral with their fight energy. They are in the fight, but you don't have to be. Honestly, it's none of your business. But you can use mental yoga to create a neutral distance between you and the couple's energy.

You can do any of these neutrality skills with your sex life. When your partner flirts with you, you can think of it as attention. Notice curiously where they touch you. Feel the sensation as you touch them with your fingertips. Stay present and neutral in your sensory body as you explore each other's lips, fingers, toes, stomachs, etc. It helps to practice neutrality out of sexual experiences first and then practice them in your sexual experiences as well.

From Neutrality to Positivity

When you've become more practiced at neutrality and sitting in the "Maybe" space on the Desire Thermometer, then you're ready to begin exploring more sex positivity and "F*ck Yes" spaces. Once you have grounded yourself in the "Maybe" space of sex, it becomes easier to play with different concepts around sex. This is when you get to rebuild new homes and resorts that are pretty, fancy and maybe even sexy. It's your neighborhood! What sexy thoughts do you want to add?

The following skills are different mental strategies that help you enjoy sex in your mind. Going from sex negativity to neutral is essentially getting to the point where you are no longer traumatized by sex or at the very least your trauma and shame are managed. Once you have gotten used to experiencing sex in neutral ways, it becomes a lot easier to go from the "Maybe" space to the yes or even "F*ck yes." These strategies include self-compassion thoughts, sexy mind games, creative sexuality, and developing a positive sexual identity.

1. Self-Compassionate Thoughts

This is where you give yourself full permission to be who you are, feel what you feel, and experience the world with kindness and compassion towards yourself. Self-compassionate thoughts sound like the words of a best friend or loving parent. When you use self-compassion regarding sex, you basically start using kind words to talk about sex or body image.

Some examples of this language come from one of my favorite yoga teachers from YouTube, Yoga with Adrienne.[37] Here are examples of her quotes. "Treat yourself like you love yourself," "Find what feels good," "Smile, just a little," "Move from a place of connect," "Inhale lots of love in, exhale lots of love out." Self-compassion thoughts impact your ability to enjoy sex and stay present in your body.

If you are trying to have an orgasm and you say things to yourself like, "It's taking so long! I hope I don't smell!", you will be drawn outside of the sexual moment. If you can say things instead that are self-compassionate like, "It's okay to take as long as you like to orgasm. It takes as long as it takes. Enjoy yourself. What's this feel like? Find what feels good," you will stay in the sexual experience and enjoy it more.

Earlier I discussed changing your mental real estate. If you dig out old sh*tty buildings, you must replace the old ones with newer nicer condos and villas that are worth living in. Otherwise, you will simply replace the old shitty houses with new shitty houses. Going from neutral to positive involves being super kind to yourself and deeply accepting who you are. Here are more examples of self-compassion language when it comes to sex and body image.

"It takes as long as it takes. Take your time. Enjoy yourself. You deserve pleasure."

"You are beautiful and worthy of love. You belong."

"You are so sexy. How dare you look this good?" ;)

"It's okay to tell (him, her, them) what you want sexually. They won't know until you tell them. It's okay to ask for your desires."

"It's okay to have desires and wants. Sex isn't only about needs. It's about passion and want. What would I like to enjoy right now?"

Self-compassion is the practice of being completely loving and accepting who you are. Embracing yourself and what you want. It involves giving yourself permission to feel sexual energy, to want or desire sexual acts or flirting, and giving yourself permission to be a sexual person. It also involves loving all your parts--your vulva, your penis, your heart, your chest, your face, your hair, your legs, your back, your breasts. It is the regular practice of deeply loving and accepting you. That, my friends, is my ultimate goal for every one of you. For more practice ideas, you can visit my YouTube channel at Youtube.com/@AngelaSkurtu and find the following videos, "How to Practice Sexual Self-Compassion,"[38] and "What is Sexual Self-Compassion?"[39]

2. Sexy Mind Games

Fantasies and daydreams are the same thing--one simply has sexual content in it. I like to teach people the skill of sexual daydreaming or fantasizing to help play in the "Maybe" space and potentially move into "yes" spaces. One important way to think about sex is that you need safety first in mind, body and context. After safety, you need excitement in mind, body, and context. So, sexual fantasies are a safe way to mentally get excited about sex.

Let's say you're watching a sex scene in a show, if you're in your "Maybe" space, you might ask, "What do you think they get out of this sexual act?" That distant question helps you engage from afar – and the best answers are in "maybes." "Maybe they get _____ out of this." There are no right or wrong answers. Give yourself permission to guess. You can break down most of sex into 3 categories-attention, connection and sensations. When you play the "Maybe Game" watching a show, try to think about what ways the couple are giving and receiving attention, creating connection, or giving and receiving sensations. Then ask yourself questions you can answer with, "Maybe we could try _____," or "Maybe if we shifted this sexual experience like _____, it could be more fun."

Next, play a game with yourself again and practice putting yourself in that sexual situation. Imagine you saw a show where they are giving a spanking. State the following, "I could be down for a spanking if _____." Inside the blank, insert any situation where you might enjoy receiving or giving a spanking. The fantasy part involves imagining yourself in that role-either the giver or the receiver. Take the fantasy beyond. Add a person you love to the story. Imagine different ways that spanking shows up.

The game is essentially, "I could be down for (insert any sexual act here) if _____." Then, fill in the blank. The sexual acts could include kissing, flirting, sensual touching, any sexual content you see on a show, any sexual content you read about, etc. Then, when you fill in the blank, think of ways to make the sexual experience fun for you. Spend time considering different situations. What are you doing? What is your partner doing? Who starts the situation? How does it start? What's a sexy way to get it started? What's a funny way to get it started? Then simply give yourself permission to play and fantasize about different things so sex starts to feel fun in your brain.

3. Learning to Embrace Creative Sexuality

Creative sexuality is stepping outside of whatever you've seen that doesn't work for you, staying in a curious space, and allowing yourself to come up with your own sexual ideas. It's a skill that gets easier with practice and helps both individuals and couples try new things. This truly involves researching sexual activities and styles that are outside the norm. For most people, a typical sexual experience includes kissing, then some touching, then oral sex, then penetrative sex. Rinse and repeat again and again. To embrace creative sexuality, you start looking at sexual expressions, acts, flirtations, and experiences that break the typical mold.

Here's how you can practice creative sexuality:

1. Think of a unique sexual act or practice (or research and find unique sexual practices).
2. Stay curious and non-judgmental.
3. Ask yourself, "If I were to do this, what's a way that it could feel good for me?"

In this process, you stay in the safety of your own fantasy in your body and mind. No one gets to tell you what to do but you. Also, you are practicing an openness to trying new things, to sexual creativity, and to exploring sex in a way that works for you.

After you practice this in your mind, you may practice it out loud with your partner. You can erotically brainstorm together ways to incorporate the sexual experience. This book is all about your personal mental relationship with sex. Stayed tuned for future books when we tackle more strategies for couples.

Grounding Yourself in Your Sexual Identity

One step in becoming more comfortable in yourself as a sexual person is to embrace your own individual sexual identity. You can think of this as making your mental real estate or "neighborhood" a *community*. You're not just rebuilding homes and resorts. You're creating a personality and a style. You're creating a warm and loving *home* inside your sexy brain.

When you think of a sexual person, who comes to mind? Typically, people will think of people like Angelina Jolie, Scarlette Johanson, Reese Witherspoon, Brad Pitt, Denzel Washington, or any other typical Hollywood sexual icon. The problem with this is they all have a similar look and feel. That's because Hollywood picks for a certain look in males and females and rarely represents people outside those roles. They tend to look young, with skinny bodies if female or muscular bodies if male. They have certain facial features and have certain ways they act if they are a sexual icon. Therein lies the problem. If you only have these narrow-minded representations of sexual identities for yourself, then if you aren't Brad Pitt, you aren't a sexual person. That's a problem for all of us!

One of the ways to embrace creative sexuality is to create your own identity as a sexual person. This may be more difficult than it sounds. To develop your own identity. Here are some questions to get you thinking about your own sexual identity:

FROM F*CK NO TO F*CK YES SEX!

How am I a sexy person? How am I different from conventional views of sexy seen in Hollywood?

What are ways they act that are different from my personal interpretation of sexy?

What actions/behaviors do they engage in that are considered sexy?

Do I consider these things sexy? Do I not? Am I somewhere in the middle?

What do I consider sexy?

When I say the word sexy, what emotions show up for me? Are they positive, neutral, painful? Where do those emotions come from?

What does the word sexy mean to me? How do I want to shift this definition?

When I show up as a sexual person, what does that look like?

For some of my clients, it can be helpful to find alternative representations of sexy people. If you are unsure what kind of sexual identity you wish to embrace, then you can start by watching shows that are counter to the typical culture of sex. Here are some examples I challenge people to watch to find their own identities: Queer Eye[40]; Lizzo Music and videos[41]; The Adams Family Movie[42]; How to Build a Sex Room[43]; any show or movie with Laverne Cox; the list can go one from there. Essentially, to develop a sexual identity that is not based on the stereotypical Hollywood look, challenge yourself to look for representation that is outside of the stereotypical box. From watching these different representations, find something that is truer to you as a person. You don't have to fit some mold. Remember spectrum thinking? Variety is the norm and eventually I hope you start to believe that variety is beautiful. Because it is. Every shape, every age, every skin color, everybody. We are meant to be a world of variety! We aren't meant to all be the same! The more we embrace variety, the easier it is to develop a sexual identity that represents you.

Your thoughts are a big deal when it comes to your sex life. It's not sex that's complicated. It's your relationship with sex that's complicated. Addressing negative thoughts is one pivotal step for enjoying sex. You can use these skills to move across the Desire Thermometer and you can learn how to do it intentionally. Start by figuring out where you are on the Desire Thermometer and move from there. The goal is to learn how to maneuver *and* how to trust yourself as you move. No one can force you to move warmer on the thermometer, but you can decide to move yourself—and then take steps towards more fun and enjoyable sex. The more you replace the old sh*tty buildings in your mind with newer, kinder or at least neutral thoughts, the better your relationship with sex will get. It's your mind. It's your real estate. You get to make it beautiful. You get to design it the way you like. Don't ever let someone else tell you how to design your brain's real estate. It's your brain and it's your home.

You can join my email list here:

OpenBedroomDoors.com

Endnotes

1. Nagoski, E. (2015). Come as you are. New York, NY: Simon and Schuster Paperbacks.

2. Wahl, D.W. (2022). "The Motivations of a Highly Critical Sexual Partner," Psychology Today, Reviewed by Tyler Woods, <https://www.psychologytoday.com/us/blog/this-sexual-self/202212/the-motivations-of-a-highly-critical-sexual-partner>

3. Nagoski, E. (2015). Come as you are. New York, NY: Simon and Schuster Paperbacks.

4. Jacobsen, J. (2024). "What is the Biggest Turn-On for Women in a Relationship?" Reviewed by Marriage.com Editorial Team, < https://www.marriage.com/advice/physical-intimacy/turn-on-for-women-in-a-relationship/>

Villines, Z. (2023). "Tips and Remedies for Getting Turned On." Medically Reviewed by Lori Lawrenz with Medical News Today. < https://www.medicalnewstoday.com/articles/how-to-get-turned-on>

5. Upham, B. (2024). "Could Embracing Body Neutrality Improve your Sex Life?" Medically Reviewed by Allison Young, M.D. with Everyday Health. < https://www.everydayhealth.com/sexual-health/could-embracing-body-neutrality-improve-your-sex-life/>

Honeycutt, F. (2022). "Opinion: Sex Neutrality is necessary for Healthy Hookup Culture." Technician Website. < https://www.technicianonline.com/opinion/opinion-sex-neutrality-is-necessary-for-healthy-hookup-culture/article_9b10f00e-4512-11ed-894f-1bd3a1012479.html#:~:text=Sex%20neutrality%20is%20the%20idea,and%20sex%20educator%2C%20Christina%20Tesoro.>

6. The Mayo Clinic Staff, "Positive Thinking: Stop Negative Self Talk to Reduce Stress." Healthy Lifestyle: Stress Management, the Mayo Clinic. Nov. 21, 2023. <https://www.mayoclinic.org/healthy-lifestyle/stress-management/in-depth/positive-thinking/art-20043950>

7. Skurtu, Angela. "How I Wish People Talked about Oral Sex." <https://www.youtube.com/watch?v=hMfKajhbtZk&t=4s>

8. "What is Exposure Therapy?" A Clinical Practice Guideline for the Treatment of PTSD. APA Division 12 (Society of Clinical Psychology). < https://www.apa.org/ptsd-guideline/patients-and-families/exposure-therapy>

9. Scott, Elizabeth (2024). "Perfectionism: 10 Signs of Perfectionist Traits: When Good Enough Isn't Enough." Reviewed by Amy Morin. Very Well Mind. June 17, 2024. <https://www.verywellmind.com/signs-you-may-be-a-perfectionist-3145233>

10. Shapiro, Jeremy. (2020) "How to Assess Black and White Thinking in Yourself and Others: Where is Your Goldilocks Zone?" Psychology Today, July 17, 2020. Review by Matt Huston. <https://www.psychologytoday.com/us/blog/thinking-in-black-white-and-gray/202007/how-assess-black-white-thinking-in-yourself-and-others>

11. National Eating Disorders Assoctiation (NEDA). <https://www.nationaleatingdisorders.org/>

12. Nagoski, E. (2015). Come as you are. New York, NY: Simon and Schuster Paperbacks.

13. Scheff, Elizabeth, (2019) "New Relationship Energy: What it is and How to Deal with it: How to sustain long-term relationships when you have a crush." Revied by Gary Drevitch, October 17, 2019, Psychology Today. < https://www.psychologytoday.com/us/blog/the-polyamorists-next-door/201910/new-relationship-energy-what-it-is-how-to-deal-with-it>

14. Grinspoon, Peter. M.D. (2022). "How to Recognize and Tame Your Cognitive Distortions." Harvard Health Publishing. Harvard Medical School. May 4, 2022. < https://www.health.harvard.edu/blog/how-to-recognize-and-tame-your-cognitive-distortions-202205042738>

15. Brown, Brene', (2014). "Why Your Critics Aren't the Ones Who Count." Youtube < https://www.youtube.com/watch?v=8-JXOnFOXQk>

16. Cote, Catherine, (2022). "Growth Mindset versus Fixed Mindset. What's the Difference?" Harvard Business School Online. March 10, 2022. < https://online.hbs.edu/blog/post/growth-mindset-vs-fixed-mindset>

17. Psychology Today Staff, (2024) Social Comparison Theory. Psychology Today. < https://www.psychologytoday.com/us/basics/social-comparison-theory>

18. Pietrangelo, Ann and Raypole, Crystal, (2023). "How to Recognize the Signs of Emotional Abuse." Healthline July 13, 2023. Reviewed by Jacquelyn Johnson, PsyD. < https://www.healthline.com/health/signs-of-mental-abuse>

19. UPMC Western Behavioral Health, (2021). "What does it Mean to Experience a Trauma Trigger?" UPMC Health Beat. August 24, 2021. < https://share.upmc.com/2021/08/trauma-trigger/>

20. https://www.youtube.com/watch?v=8Siah5R44FQ&t=3s

21. The Editors of Encyclopaedia Britannica, (2025) "Sympathetic Nervous System: Anatomy." Last Updated January 7, 2025. Britannica Website. < https://www.britannica.com/science/neurotransmitter>

22. Maltz, W. (2012). The sexual healing journey: a guide for survivors of sexual abuse. ; Chicago / Turabian - Author Date Citation · Maltz, Wendy.

23. "**Healing Sex**. A Mind-Body Approach to Healing Sexual Trauma". By **Staci Haines**. San Francisco: Cleis Press, 2007. 266 pages, $25.95 (paperback).

24. Shershun, Erica (2021). Healing Sexual Trauma Workbook: Somatic Skills to Help you Feel Safe in Your Body, Create Boundaries, and Live with Resilience." New Harbinger Publications.

25. https://www.youtube.com/watch?v=goS7jhsKrRg&t=31s

26. Stinson, Adrienne (2024). "What is Box Breathing?" Medically reviewed by Timothy J. Legg. Medical News Today, Updated May 13th, 2024. < https://www.medicalnewstoday.com/articles/321805>

27. Xie, Weiyang, (2018). "Dare to Rewire your Brain for Self Compassion." TedXUnd April 2018. < https://www.ted.com/talks/weiyang_xie_dare_to_rewire_your_brain_for_self_compassion>

28. Yoda, (1980). "Star Wars: The Empire Strikes Back." Director Irvin Kershner, LucasFilm, LTD.

29. Silverberg, Cory. (2015) "Sex is a Funny Word: A Book about Bodies, Feelings, and You." Triangle Square Publishing.

30. Michaels, L., Fey, T., Waters, M.S., Lohan, L., (2009). *Mean Girls*. Paramount.

31. Millard, E. (2023) "Body Neutrality: How trading affirmation for acceptance can be freeing." Experience Life, June 2023. Pp. 56-61.

32. Millard, E. (2023) "Body Neutrality: How trading affirmation for acceptance can be freeing." Experience Life, June 2023. Pp. 56-61. < https://experiencelife.lifetime.life/article/what-is-body-neutrality-and-how-can-i-embrace-it/>

33. Mind Charity in England. "Mindfulness." November 2021. < https://www.mind.org.uk/information-support/drugs-and-treatments/mindfulness/about-mindfulness/>

34. McCartney, J. (2006). "The Great Wall of Vulva," Art of England. < https://www.thegreatwallofvulva.com/>

35. < https://www.youtube.com/watch?v=e_H5z7TWpMM&t=170s>

36. < https://www.youtube.com/watch?v=WoblZb9y_Ik&t=12s>

37. Mishler, A. < https://www.youtube.com/user/yogawithadriene>

38. < https://www.youtube.com/watch?v=9sIYCx_uGCE&t=66s>

39. < https://www.youtube.com/watch?v=fA0y8Rpmcak&t=42s>

40. Collins, D. (2018 t0 Present). Queer Eye Tv Series. Netflix.

41. Lizzo. American rapper and singer. <https://www.lizzomusic.com/>

42. Sonnonfield, (1991). The Adams Family. Paramount Picture and Orion Pictures.

43. Rose, M. (2022). How to Build a Sex Room TV Series. Netflix.

"As one of the brightest voices in the sex therapy world, Angela Skurtu has written an easy to follow, practical, and compassionate guide to improving your sex life. Her expertise shines in this volume with the engaging voice of a knowledgeable friend who wants to and will help you to have to best sex you can!"

Greyson Smith, MA, LPC - Couples and Sex Therapist

"It's *not* what you think. It's not about positions or sex toys. It helps you change the way you think about sex. It's good for dating and marriage. I've learned so much about myself reading this book!"

Anoynmous, Friend, Editor, and Beta Reader

About the Illustrator

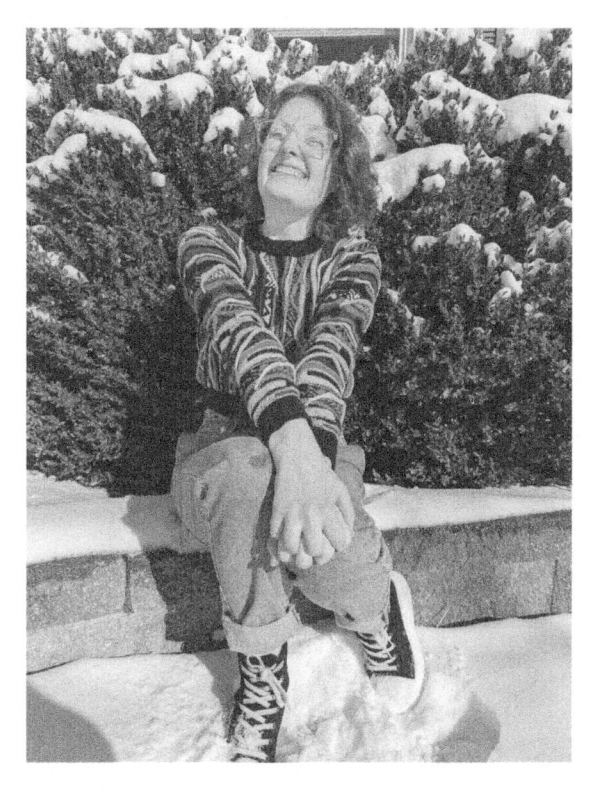

Whitney Stubblefield a funny woman with a talent for art. She graduated with a BFA in Fine Arts and is eager to make her mark in the world. You can often find her doodling some kind of weird alien or sexy graphic art at her desk at home. Whitney is a graphic designer willing to create graphic art for anyone who wants to put their thoughts into an image. You can find her at whitneyrstubblefield@gmail.com if you want to hire her to make graphic art for your books or website.

About the Author

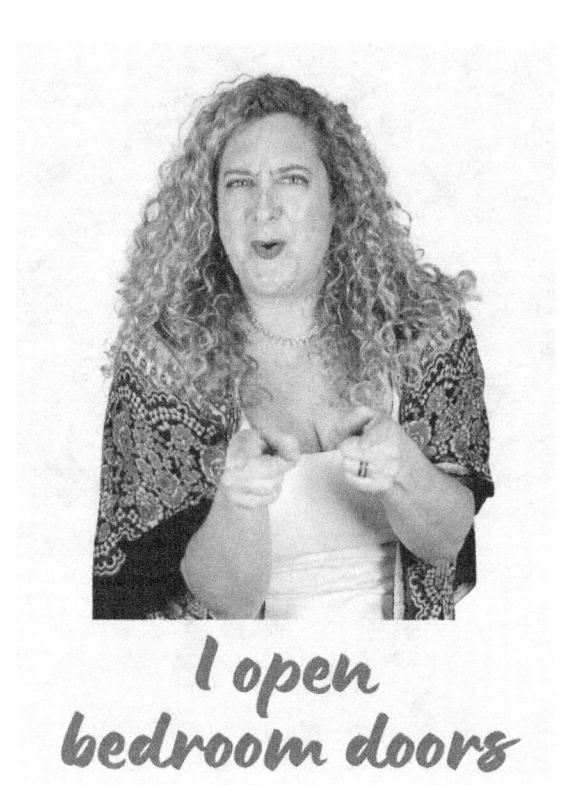

I open bedroom doors

Angela Skurtu, M.Ed., LMFT, CST. Angela is a Keynote Speaker and Author of the books Pre-Marital Counseling: A Guide for Clinicians (2016), Helping Couples Overcome Infidelity: A Therapist's Manual (2018). She is a Licensed Marriage Therapist and Supervisor in the state of Missouri (AAMFT) and an Certified Sex Therapist and Supervisor (AASECT). Angela Skurtu also has a YouTube channel Youtube.com/c/angelaskurtu and upcoming podcast where she offers free relationship and sexual health skills.

Angela Skurtu on a personal level: I love this work. Every day, I am privileged to walk with couples in their time of need and help sexually empower them. For many of the couples I work with, sex is mired in shame. Instead of feeling comfortable in their body, sex is scary, lonely, and creates anxiety. My work with couples is all about helping them find their own creative sexual style and become their authentic sexual selves. When someone comes to me and says, "I am not a sexual person," that has more to do with what society has taught them about what it means to be sexual then who they actually are as a sexual person. My passion is to help individuals find their sexual voice and their personal sexual identity. I'm Angela Skurtu and **I open bedroom doors!**

For more information about Angela's products and to join her email list, go to Openbedroomdoors.com and submit a contact form.

About the "Open Bedroom Doors" Book Series

Recently, I was reading an age-appropriate sex education book to my 10-year-old daughter. She asked me, "Is naked sexy?" My face broke out into a sweat. I thought to myself, *how do I answer this question in a way a 10-year-old can understand? I'm a sex therapist. I talk to adults about this all the time! What in the world do I say to her?*

I awkwardly answered, "Well, honey, not all naked is sexy. Sometimes naked is for fun. Sometimes it's sexy. Sometimes it's just what you need to do." She looked at me puzzled. I got up to demonstrate.

"Sometimes, it's fun," I said as I danced around in a silly way. She laughed and danced with me. She had just gotten out of the bath.

"Sometimes, it's sexy," then I playfully tried to show her how a sexy person might pose. Imagine an awkward mom trying out one of those Swimsuit edition magazine poses with the puffy lips and the bedroom eyes. *Nailed it!*

"Sometimes, it's just what you need to do. Like right now, you just got out of the bath. You had to be naked for your bath and now we're going to get you into PJs for bed," she and I laughed, and I thought, *phew, problem solved.*

Later that week, a similar conversation came up with a 40-year-old client. A woman was sitting in my office. We discussed using nudity as a way to build intimacy with her partner.

"You could have a naked TV night," I suggested. She stared at me terrified. Her face grew white. "I'm not suggesting you have sex *every* time you're naked. Like, you could just sit and cuddle naked watching a fun show." I thought to myself, *what just happened here?*

"Wait, it's not about sex?" she asked, bewildered.

"Well, it *can* be, but it doesn't *have* to be," I responded. "Let me explain like I just taught my daughter this week." At that point, I got up and did the exact same lesson I gave my daughter. I got up and acted playful, sexy and then neutrally. "You see? You can do all kinds of things naked. It *can* be sexy, but it doesn't *have* to be sexy." I thought to myself, *I hope she understood.*

Then it hit me, this woman is avoiding sex because she doesn't know there are options for how she can be intimate with her partner. This couple is in a sexless marriage because they never learned how to talk about sex and set boundaries around it so it can be fun. They need creative sexuality!

I'm writing the *Open Bedroom Doors* book series because many of you have unhealthy relationships with sex. It's not sex that's complicated, it's your *relationship* with sex that's complicated. Sex education is actually **abuse prevention**. When you teach kids how to own and honor their bodies at a young age, you teach them how to set boundaries for themselves and advocate for themselves in future sexual situations. In this book series I am teaching adults the sex education they never received as children.

That is the problem. Most of us had little or no sex education. As a result, you got into sexual situations and didn't know what you were doing. Some of you faired okay. But many of you ended up in painful situations that could have been prevented with healthy, comprehensive, medically accurate sex education. Most of you learned through trial by fire. FYI, sex can be a *very* hot fire and leave you with third degree burns. Every day, I walk with couples and individuals who have been sexually *burned* and it could have been prevented.

I can't let this happen anymore. I plan to reparent the nation one book at a time. The *Open Bedroom Doors* book series will teach adults the sex education they never received as kids. It will cover ways to talk to your kids about sex. It will cover senior sex. It will cover sexual transitions like finding yourself after a divorce. It will cover ways to change your relationship with sex. It will support you in finding a healthier future journey with sex. This book is only the beginning. Stay tuned!

Join my email list at Openbedroomdoors.com

Made in the USA
Monee, IL
17 March 2025